INTERMITTENT FASTING AND KETOGENIC DIET:

How to Use ~~_____~~
Adapt ~~_____~~ *t,*

D1435235

... McCampbell

Legal & Disclaimer

The information contained in this book is not designed to replace or take the place of any form of medicine or professional medical advice. The information in this book has been provided for educational and entertainment purposes only. The information contained in this book has been compiled from sources deemed reliable, and it is accurate to the best of the Author's knowledge; however, the Author cannot guarantee its accuracy and validity and cannot be held liable for any errors or omissions. Changes are periodically made to this book. You must consult your doctor or get professional medical advice before using any of the suggested remedies, techniques, or information in this book.

Upon using the information contained in this book, you agree to hold harmless the Author from and against any damages, costs, and expenses, including any legal fees potentially resulting from the application of any of the information provided by this guide. This disclaimer applies to any damages or injury caused by the use and application, whether directly or indirectly, of any advice or information presented, whether for breach of contract, tort, negligence, personal injury, criminal intent, or under any other cause of action.

You agree to accept all risks of using the information presented inside this book. You need to consult a professional medical practitioner in order to ensure you are both able and healthy enough to participate in this program.

Table of Contents

Introduction

If you're looking to lose weight but not muscle, let this be your guide to a new lifestyle, with a complete revision of your dietary intake. This book is not about a specific diet that you just know you can't stick to because of those cravings. It is about a whole new way of eating.

Intermittent Fasting (IF) is a quick means of putting the body into ketosis. That may sound a little unnerving, but in fact, it is a natural state for the body to be in. In this guide, I will show you exactly what IF means, and how to go about it as a regular part of your life. It is simply a case of permanently changing the way you eat.

With an IF plan, you can eat anything you like in your eating windows, but I recommend sticking to healthy meals. Foods high in carbs, sugar and salt have shown to cause cravings, the results of which will make it more difficult to stick to a healthy eating regime. We all know that takeout and store-bought processed foods are high in sugars and salts - ingredients that are unhealthy for your overall wellbeing. There would be little point in introducing IF into your life if you kept eating unhealthily and gaining excess weight.

It is sensible to eat healthy foods, no matter what your personal dietary routine is. That's why I would like to show you how eating low-carb ingredients will enhance all your efforts whilst using IF. A low-carb dietary intake will help you lose excess stored fat while maintaining important muscle bulk. I personally chose the ketogenic (keto) diet for myself, which is why I use it in this book. I believe everyday life should be about maintaining healthy eating habits as well as losing and keeping off any unwanted excess weight.

This is a book about healthy eating habits and introducing IF into your daily life. To understand this concept, I will show you:

- **How to start IF, and all the different ways you can do it.**

- **What happens to your body when it is in ketosis.**

- **The good and the bad effects of ketosis.**

- **How to distinguish good and bad fats.**

- **How to measure your food intake with macronutrients.**

- **Meal suggestions.**

- **Plus a few easy exercises to help tone up the muscle in your body while losing weight.**

Not only are IF and a low-carb keto diet good for your weight but also your overall health. Benefits include:

- **Decreasing your chances of cardiovascular diseases.**

- **Decreasing your chances of certain cancers.**

- **Preserving the leanness in your body mass with increased Human Growth Hormones (HGH).**

- **Improving concentration skills.**

If you want to lose weight, feel good, and stay fit, then read on.

Thank you so much for your support through buying and reading this book, it means the world to me!

If you never want to miss out on one of my future books, consider signing up for my newsletter here

http://bit.ly/allannewsletter

and checking out my author's page here

http://amzn.to/allanmccampbell

Chapter 1 - What Is Intermittent Fasting (IF)?

Most people who use Intermittent Fasting (IF) are doing so to try and lose excess weight (burning off fat that is in storage).

I will begin by explaining what happens to the body during the "fasting state."

In the following chapters, I will show you different ways of using the IF method, but first you need to have a little understanding of what it's all about.

By using IF, you are not necessarily dieting. This is because during eating periods you can eat anything you like, although it is advisable to eat healthy foods. You do not need to restrict your calorie count during the eating periods if you don't wish to. However, in this book, I will be looking at using the keto diet in conjunction with IF. Dietary control is not necessary with IF if you don't want to do that.

By itself, IF is simply a means of introducing a new routine of eating. It's an alternative routine that can replace the traditional 3-4 meals a day. There are various methods to do IF, such as missing meals or fasting for longer periods. Don't worry, IF is only undertaken in small steps, so you will not starve, but more about that later.

Insulin

The "Eating Period" or "Fed State" means that while you are eating, and around 4hrs afterwards, your body's insulin levels are at their highest. Insulin is a hormone. One of its tasks is to trigger the liver to take glucose from the bloodstream and store it for energy later. There are many other uses for insulin, which shows what an important hormone it is, given it functions correctly. When those fat reserves are not used because the body is not burning enough energy to dip into the reserves, it results in an increase in weight.

Burning Excess Fat

It will be another 10-12 hours after a meal before your body enters the "fasted state." This is when the body will begin to burn the excess reserves of fat. It stands to reason then, that if you are eating regular meals and not burning enough energy, you are never going to reach the fat burning stage.

Should you choose to use IF as a part of your dietary control, you will find that you will not yearn for any particular foods, as none are banned. If you skip a meal, it is not simply the lack of calories that will help you lose weight. It is rather that your body takes its energy from the excess fat stores. This is because you are not producing that all-important glucose (sugary energy) as you are in the "fasted state."

Muscle Mass

Stored fat is burned up before muscle fat, so it is unlikely that you will lose weight in muscle mass when you fast.

Other Benefits of IF

Clinical trials of animals on IF show:

- **Chronic Disease - During the "fasted state", there was a decreased risk of any signs of chronic diseases.**

- **Diabetes - There were signs of lower diabetes incidents due to lowered glucose and insulin concentrations.**

- **Cardiovascular - Cholesterol levels and heart rates lowered. This means they had less risk of any type of cardiovascular disease.**

- **Cancer - Certain cancerous cells decreased, with a reduction in lymphoma occurrences. Better survival rates, even with tumors, have been proven.**

- **Human Growth Hormones (HGH) - We produce these mostly while we sleep. Fasting is also a good stimulus for increasing HGH levels. The result of this is the preservation of lean mass.**

Chapter 2 - Ways of Intermittent Fasting

Now that I've explained the basics of Intermittent Fasting, let's move forward and see how it's done. There are different ways of achieving good results through IF.

Before I discuss the various ways of IF, there is some amazing positive feedback out there for this dietary regime. You will find people who have been successful with this method and swear by it. Most appear to agree that it is an easier way to lose weight than sticking to a specific diet. This is because you don't need to stick to particular foodstuff as long as you choose healthy ingredients. The consensus among people seems to be that it's more of a routine than an actual diet. Once you're used to that routine, you will do it automatically.

That said, let's consider the different methods. Then you can decide which one would suit your lifestyle.

The main choices are either skipping meals or having fasting days. Either way will have the same effect on your metabolism. When done correctly, both will lead you to the stage where your body starts to burn up fat resources after hours of not eating.

There are 6 different ways of reaching ketosis. By understanding them, you can decide which is best for you:

Eating Window - Leangain

- Within a 24hr period, you have an eating window of up to 8hrs. This means that you can eat whatever you want, whenever you want, though it's still better to make healthy choices.

- One way of achieving this is to eat nothing after your evening meal and then skip breakfast altogether.

- For this method, you need to fast for 16hrs.

- If you like your breakfast, this may not be the right method for you.

- Popular eating windows are: 18/6; 20/4; 21/3. The lower numbers equal how many hours you have to eat within. Pick which one suits you and your lifestyle the best.

- This is done daily and becomes a routine, though you do not have to do it daily if you don't like the sound of that. Try it for a week on, then a week off.

2 Day Fasting - 5/2

- For any 5 days of the week, you will eat the normal 3 meals, choosing healthy ingredients.

- The other two days are for fasting.

- This method is slightly different in that you can eat during the fasting period, but you must limit the total calorie intake to 500 on each fasting day.

- For the best results, do not have the fasting days consecutively.

Alternate Days

- This means fasting every other day.

- If this sounds unachievable, some people allow themselves 500 calories on fasting days.

24hr

- Fasting for 24hrs once or twice a week (not on consecutive days).

- The 24hr period begins when you have your last meal, for instance from breakfast to breakfast.

Missing Meals

- Skip a meal every now and then.

- Good for those who don't like breakfast, as they can easily skip it every day.

- Or skip lunch every day.

Day V Night

- During the day, you only eat raw fruit or raw vegetables.

- At night, you will have one main meal.

How to Get Started

- Some of these methods can be quite difficult to achieve for a beginner. So, if that's you, decide which is the best way to get started with a new dietary regime!

- It might be best to start gently, for example by missing the occasional meal as per option 5. Try this for a month and see if it works for you.

- This will let you know how your body feels when missing out on a meal.

- Once you're into the routine, move on to skipping 1 meal a day every day, such as breakfast or lunch.

- You may then feel ready to look at doing one of the longer fasting methods, whereby you will need to fast for several hours at a time.

- Note that when you are fasting, you can still drink fluids such as water, tea and coffee, although it's best to skip the milk in warm drinks. It is important to drink plenty of liquids to avoid dehydration.

- Drinking will also help with feelings of hunger.

- You will experience cravings once you begin to fast for longer hours, but they are not permanent. They will come at you in waves rather than be there all the time.

- It also helps if you can keep busy and not think about being hungry.

- Try not to overindulge after a fasting period.

- It's important to eat healthily when not fasting. No binge-eating or fast food takeout.

- Just as you would start your day with a small breakfast, the same rule applies after forced fasting. When you finish a fasting period, start with a small meal.

This last statement nicely leads us to the second topic of this book. You have learned about fasting, what happens to your body and how to go about it. Let's have a look at the best food ingredients to help achieve your goals. Our next few chapters are going to look at the ketogenic diet, which compliments IF perfectly.

Chapter 3 - Metabolic State of Ketosis

Most of us realize that sugary carbohydrates are unhealthy, especially when eaten in excess. Usually, they are only beneficial before a workout or an activity that will burn a lot of energy. Our body uses carbs for energy. If you eat more energy than you burn, those carbs are stored away as fat, for use at a later time.

Therefore, it makes sense to change your dietary intake to include more low-carb foodstuff. A keto diet is about consuming high-fat, medium-protein and low-carb foods. Don't be put off by the words "high-fat" because it is "good" fat that you will be consuming.

Putting that aside for a moment, let's have a look at what the metabolic state of "ketosis" actually means.

Ketosis and Ketones

Most importantly, ketosis is not an unnatural state for your body to be in. If food was in short supply, your body would automatically enter the metabolic state of ketosis to survive. This means that your body is using fat instead of sugar to find its energy.

What is Ketosis?

- Ketosis is a metabolic process.

- Carbs turn into sugar, known as glucose, in the bloodstream. The hormone known as insulin processes that sugar into energy. If it cannot find any glucose, here's what will happen in your body:

- Insulin levels will drop because it is not needed.

- For its energy source, your body will begin to burn up the body fat that is in storage.

- It is now burning fat instead of glucose.

- Your body is now in the metabolic state of "ketosis."

Why is Ketosis Beneficial?
- Diabetes

When the insulin levels drop in ketosis, the blood sugars are naturally lowered. This also regulates the high spiking of blood sugars. It is a great way to help people with Type II Diabetes balance their blood sugar levels.

- Losing Weight

If you are too heavy for your size, chances are that you are eating too many carbs. Most of that glucose in your bloodstream will be stored away for later use. The result of this is excess body mass. Eating low-carb food means that your body will naturally begin to burn that excess body fat.

- Coronary Disease

Triglycerides - Body fat consists of triglycerides. These are components of a sugar alcohol called Glycerol, plus the fatty acids that stick to it. As this is all a part of our metabolic status, it can be measured. If it is too high or too low, then your health is at risk. Too high has a similar effect as a high cholesterol count and means that you are more at risk for coronary heart disease. A normal count would come in at around 150. Ketosis lowers the triglyceride levels, so you are less at risk for coronary diseases.

Cholesterol - This is a fatty substance within a cell. It is also known as Lipids. Because it is oil-based, it floats around the water-based bloodstream. Again, this can be measured in a few ways. If you have a high level of Low-Density Lipoprotein (LDL), it is means you are more at risk for coronary heart disease.

Ketosis helps to balance both Triglycerides and Cholesterol levels to a healthier state. Eating foods high in healthy fats helps to produce High-Density Lipoprotein (HDL). At the same time it lowers Low-Density Lipoprotein (LDL) in your cholesterol levels. These are the bad fats. A keto diet has proven to improve the makeup of Triglycerides levels. The result of this is lower blood pressure and less risk for coronary diseases.

- Clearer Concentration

An organelle called a mitochondrion is something you produce in your cells. It turns nutrients into energy or glucose within each cell.

A molecule known as a "Free Radical" is also produced in our cells. These help us to fight off bacteria and viruses. Sometimes these are overproduced, and that makes us ill.

A higher mitochondrial rate in your cells lowers the production of Free Radicals, which is good, as they can hamper cell function.

A keto diet increases the mitochondrial rate, which helps to increase energy levels and clear our minds for better focus.

These are but a few examples of health benefits from a keto diet. It can take a few days for your body to enter ketosis, as you will be burning up any sugars that are still present in the bloodstream.

In my next chapter I will compare some of the negative implications of being in the metabolic state of ketosis.

Chapter 4 - Can Ketosis Be Harmful?

There is still much to debate on this matter.

Because ketosis is a natural state, some believe it cannot harm the body or the organs.

When your body has been in ketosis for a long time, you can go into ketoacidosis.

This condition, known as Diabetic Ketoacidosis (DKA), is harmful for a diabetic. It means that glucose levels are too high and insulin levels too low. This is a typical condition in Diabetes Type I. The patient must seek immediate help to raise insulin levels and reduce the amount of sugar in the blood.

On a keto diet, you can control ketoacidosis. When you stay in ketosis for too long, the lack of sugar in the bloodstream lowers the insulin levels, sometimes to a harmful level. Combined with the lack of glucose in the bloodstream, this causes an increased presence of acids known as ketones. You can measure your ketone levels by using urine test strips.

- The normal level of ketones is 0.6 mmol/L.

- When on a keto diet, your reading will be higher but should not go over 1.5 mmol/L.

- Anything above 1.6 mmol/L means your ketone levels are too high and you must take action.

- Drink plenty of water to flush out the ketones from your system, as you need to rehydrate your body.

- Include more carbs in your diet for a day and take your body out of ketosis.

- You can go back into it once your keto levels have been at a normal level for a short while.

Many people spend years in the state of ketosis without any side effects. There simply is not enough evidence to say it is harmful for everyone. Ketosis affects people differently.

Here's a few signs to look out for that may indicate your body is not coping well in ketosis. If you have any of these symptoms, then it's time to test your urine and maybe come out of ketosis for a short while. For some, these symptoms only occur when the body first enters the state of ketosis and go away as it adjusts:

- Bad Breath - You may know it as keto-breath because is it unique to the state of ketosis. The ketones that are building up in your bloodstream are now exiting your body through your breath, urine and sweat. You may experience a metallic taste in your mouth. This signals the buildup of Acetone, a chemical produced by your body.

- Body Salts - There will be an imbalance in your bodily fluids, as salts may get flushed out more than normally. It is imperative to maintain your hydration levels. If you start to suffer headaches, this could be because you are dehydrated and have a high loss of body salts. The body's natural electrolytes, such as potassium and magnesium, may also suffer temporarily, resulting in body cramps. By increasing certain foods, you can soon get back that balance and maintain it.

- Keto Flu – Unfortunately, there is a transitional period known as keto adaption during which your body adjusts to ketosis. This can take a few weeks in the beginning. You may experience food cravings, fatigue, insomnia, dizziness and lack of concentration. Your heart may feel like it's racing at times, but it's all a part of keto adaption. What you eat will play an important part in how it affects you. I will discuss dietary intake of low-carb, high-fat and medium-protein foods later in the book.

- Digestive System - Everything you do in life seems to influence your bowels, and keto adaption is no different. It could also be the different foods you are now eating more of that are causing troubles in your digestive system. When I discuss the keto dietary intake, I'll show you the best way of dealing with problems such as constipation.

It may all sound a little worrying and make you wonder if it is worth doing. People who are on low-carb diets with Intermittent Fasting often say it is just a change of lifestyle and not a fixed diet. The health benefits are good so long as you do it right. That way you can avoid or at least cut down on any of the negative effects of ketosis.

I've looked at the Good, the Bad, and the downright Ugly aspects of ketosis. Let's now consider what types of foods you would need to include in your daily dietary intake in order to experience more of the Good.

Chapter 5 - Is Low Carb Eating Bad for You?

I have already discussed the possible negative side effects of ketosis. It is also important to understand what difficulties your body may experience when you start cutting down on the carbs. Don't let the following symptoms put you off - I mention them purely for educational purposes. Ideally, this should not be a temporary diet but become a way of life. You may want to take a time out from the fasting regime, but you should keep up the low-carb dietary intake. Eventually, those sugar and carb cravings will stop, especially as you slowly increase your carb intake again. When you first embark upon this new eating regime, there will be changes going on in your body as it adjusts.

What bad effects can you expect in the beginning when reducing your carbohydrate intake?

Lacking Fiber

This is a possibility, especially in the beginning as you will be cutting out food types such as grains and wheat. Some foods that you ate for fiber, for your digestive system, will be a no-go area. Constipation could become an issue if you are not careful, so it's important to continue eating fiber. When low-carbing, you should be getting your fiber from non-starchy vegetables such as:

- Leafy greens like kale and spinach

- Broccoli and cauliflower

- Nuts

- Berries

➔ Try sprinkling 1 tbsp. flax seed over some of your meals. Once mixed in, you'll hardly even know it's there.

➔ Walking is a good way to get the bowels moving naturally. Increase your cardiac exercises; they help more than just your heart.

Dehydration

- If you don't drink enough water to soak in the extra fiber you are eating, you may suffer terrible flatulence and make the constipation worse.

- Ensure you drink plenty of fluids to avoid these problems.

Too Much Protein

- Since you will be eating more foods that are high in protein, you need to be aware that your kidney and liver will be working harder.

- If you already suffer any health problems in these areas, perhaps a low-carb diet is not right for you.

- The increased protein consumption could cause you to pass higher concentrations of calcium in your urine, which can lead to kidney stones.

- Your protein intake is supposed to be medium, but eating more meat to increase fat intake might create an imbalance.

Affecting Metabolism and Thyroid Function

I've talked about electrolytes such as magnesium during ketosis. As you begin this low-carb way of eating, other changes could be happening inside your body:

- The thyroids produce natural hormones such as triiodothyronine (T3). There is going to be a hormonal imbalance once ketosis kicks in. Hormonal imbalances can lead to mood swings, sluggishness and difficulty in concentration.

- This can cause changes in your immune system, as low T3 levels slow down your metabolism rates, which then leads to weight gain.

- Studies have also shown that this can result in lower testosterone levels, which, in turn, can lead to a low libido.

- There can also be an increase of the natural steroid cortisol levels, which can cause cravings and increase blood sugar levels.

Therefore, it's important not to cut down on the calorie intake. Keep your dietary intake at a nutritious level and don't be sedentary. Cutting carbs should not cause any thyroid intolerance if you are eating healthily. You also need to be performing basic exercises at the very least. This way, you should naturally increase the important hormone T3 levels.

All this raises the question: Should you take supplements?

It is safe to say that natural supplements such as omega 3 are always good to take. As mentioned, your dietary intake should include nutritious foods. If you have a good nutritional balance, you normally shouldn't require supplements. At the start of the keto diet you might become aware of a few unpleasant changes (as discussed in Chapter 4). In that case, it might help to add daily supplements to support your new regime, such as:

Fish Oil

- Sodium, potassium and magnesium levels may decline, so you could consider organic supplements.

- Alternatively, eat plenty of foods that will give you a natural supply, such as spinach and kale, tomatoes, avocados, blackberries, cheese, yogurt, nuts, fish, dark chocolate and even bananas.

- You can take tests at home to check your electrolyte levels and keep an eye on them.

Vitamin D

- The body produces vitamin D when the skin is exposed to sunlight. If there's not much sunshine around, you may benefit from using a supplement.

- This vitamin helps the bones to absorb calcium for strength and boosts the immune system.

If you want to take supplements, choose organic ones without added sugar.

Multivitamins combine multiple vitamins, which would eliminate the need to take several different ones.

Follow the directions on the label and don't overdose on any supplements.

Better still, sit down and make meal plans. This way, you know you are going to get a good mixed range of natural nutritional foods. If you do it right, you should not need to take supplements. Therefore, it's worth taking the time to plan ahead in order to avoid any of the symptoms I have talked about in this chapter.

Chapter 6 - Foods to Eat on a Ketogenic Diet

The keto diet is similar to the Atkins diet because both limit carb intake. As previously mentioned, the foods you eat are going to put your body into ketosis. Ingredients for meals I'm going to mention in this chapter will be:

- Low-carb
- High-fat (good fats)
- Medium-protein

In this book, I'll be focusing on Intermittent Fasting (IF) combined with the keto diet. This means that once you've chosen which method of fasting is best for you, your eating windows will include keto food. As I've already discussed, fasting is a quick way for the body to enter ketosis. It's still important to make sure that when you are eating, you are complimenting the fasting efforts with the right types of food.

The whole point of the keto diet is to enter ketosis. IF will get you to that stage quicker:

- Using the IF method to enter ketosis results in fewer bad side effects.

- Putting yourself on a keto diet makes ketosis easier to handle. That's because when you are eating, you are not coming in and out of ketosis but staying in it.

- Plus, the keto is a high-fat diet, which helps curbing appetite. When you do eat, you will eat less.

- During your eating window, you should stick to IF-recommended foods rather than load up on carbs.

Now, you can see that Intermittent Fasting and ketogenic dieting go hand in hand.

Fats on a Keto Diet

As this is a high-fat diet, you must ensure you eat foods with good fats. Look for the following types of fats in your food:
- Saturated (in moderation)
- Monounsaturated (helps to raise good cholesterol levels)

- Polyunsaturated

Avoid:
- Trans fats
- Hydrogenated fats

To find out more about fats, see the chapter on Good and Bad Fats, but for now let's move on to the food ingredients.

Food Types on a Keto Diet

- Fats - Eat fats that come from natural sources such as nuts, seeds, and red meat.
- Protein - Lean meats, white meats, and dairy products.
- Vegetables - The more the better, and they don't have to be fresh – frozen ones are just as effective.
- Water - It is essential to stay hydrated. Any liquid is fine, so long as it's not laced with sugar.
- Note that there are no sugary foods on the list. It's recommended that you keep your carb levels to around 30-50 net grams a day. You can still eat fruit, but make sure you deduct the natural sugars from your daily carb intake.

- If you adjust your body to eating low-carb, you may at first crave to eat more food. Eventually, the high-fat foods will fill you, and the cravings will pass. Try to stick to non-starch vegetables such as greens rather than potatoes or squashes. Starchy vegetables do have carbs, so account for that in your daily allowance.

Summary of food list on a keto diet:

GOOD

- Lean meats and offal (particularly grass-fed as this produces more omega 3)

- Oily fish, red salmon, mackerel, sardines, trout, herring, anchovies, bass, bod, halibut, pollack, and canned tuna (Oily fish is high in omega 3)

- Non-carb shellfish such as crab, shrimp, or crawfish

- Vegetables: Non-starchy greens such as cabbage, kale, spinach, broccoli, Brussel sprouts, chard, chives, soy leaves, lettuce, cucumber, zucchini, bamboo shoots, and asparagus

- Dairy: Eggs, cheeses, and butter

- Oil: Coconut, and extra virgin olive

- Fruit: Olives without fillings

- Miscellaneous: Shirataki noodles, tea and coffee with no sugar or milk (if you need milk, you should use full fat or cream), natural herbs and spices

MIDDLE - With Low Carb Content

- Lean meats and offal (Grain-fed)

- Fish: Tuna steaks, pink salmon, flounder, haddock, and pike

- Shellfish: Clams, lobster, mussels, and scallops

- Vegetables: starchy veg, such as root vegetables, mushrooms, onions, peppers, eggplant, peas, tomatoes, or artichoke

- Dairy: Always choose full-fat - plain yogurts, or cream

- Oil: Vegetable oils

- Fruit: Berries, avocado, coconut, pears, apples, and peaches

- Miscellaneous: Red wine, unsweetened spirits, nuts and seeds, dark chocolate, soy sauce, soy beans, and sweeteners (could cause cravings)

AVOID

- Low-fat products

- Processed foods

- Sugars

- Factory-farmed meat

- Grains

- Beans and Legumes

- Beers and Ales or any sweetened alcohol, fresh juices, and sodas

- Sugary foods

- Certain fruits such as most tropical fruits, bananas, honeydew melon, figs and dates, papayas, pineapple, mango, and dried fruits

- High starch vegetables such as white or red potatoes

Chapter 7 - What Are Good Fats and Bad Fats?

If you care about what you eat, then you may be aware that there is much confusion on this topic. In the past, food and medical experts warned us that too much fat in the diet was detrimental to our health. Now, we have all learned that much of that advice appears to have been misleading. The human body needs a certain amount of fat to function correctly. Just as it needs salt in moderation. When you're conscientious about what you eat, it can be a minefield of what to believe. This chapter should clear up some myths about fat.

Low Fat Dietary Intake

The word "fat" alone sounds unpleasant. That's because in the media, it is often linked to an unhealthy lifestyle and obesity. We all need to watch the amount of fat content in our diet. Surprisingly, not only is too much bad for us, but too little also has health implications.

Too little fat in your diet can result in:

- Being unable to absorb natural fat soluble vitamins, such as A, D, K and E. Such vitamins are essential for the immune system, blood clotting and growth. With insufficient fat in your diet, these vitamins are more likely to be expelled from the body as waste. This is because fat helps to absorb them into the bloodstream.

- Studies have indicated that those who have insufficient fat in their diets are more susceptible to mental illnesses and mood swings. That includes conditions such as bipolar disorder and schizophrenia. It does not stop there as it also includes eating disorders like bulimia and anorexia. It is therefore best to include essential fatty acids in your daily meal plan such as omega 3 and omega 6, which are found in nuts, seeds, oils, beans and fruits.

- Certain cancers, such as prostrate, colon and breast. Increasing omega 3 and omega 6 will help the body slow down cancer cell growth.

- An increased risk of heart disease. Many on a low-fat diet crave carbohydrates thereby risking to eat more unhealthy foodstuff. In turn, this increases the risk of cardiovascular disease. Those who have a diet high in the good fats have a lower mortality rate.

- Overeating, as you will not have the "feel full" effect. Fats help enhancing flavor and make us feel full for longer.

- The risks of low-fat diets have a similar effect to eating too much of the wrong fats. This proves that a good balance of fats is essential to you daily dietary intake.

Molecular Groupings of Fat

There are three main types of Carbon Chain Fatty Acids:
- SCFA or SCTs - Short Chain Fatty Acids
- MCFA or MCTs - Medium Chain Fatty Acids
- LCFA or LCTs - Long Chain Fatty Acids

Fatty Acids are the glycerol molecules (sugar liquids) that are made up of chains of hydrogen atoms.

Hydrogen Atoms refer to atoms that gel everything together.

Triglycerides are fatty acid carbon atoms, also joined together by hydrogen atoms.

The combination of these molecules is how we can decipher if the fat is good or bad for us.

Let's now break up the lengths of Triglyceride chains:

- Saturated fat: no more than 2 hydrogen atoms joined to each carbon atom
- Monounsaturated fat: no hydrogen atoms at all
- Polyunsaturated fat: some missing hydrogen atoms

The more hydrogen atoms are missing to join the carbon atoms together, the weaker the chain link becomes. This is when the fat gets bad for your health.

Which foods have which fats?

- SCTs: found in leafy greens and grains such as buckwheat
- MCTs: found in dairy products and coconut oil
- LCTs: found in olive oil, fish and nuts

MCTs

Foods high in MCTs are ideal when on a ketogenic diet. These fats have the capability to stabilize sugar levels in the blood. MCTs travel straight to the liver, where they are turned into ketones. This process serves as an energy source without raising blood sugar levels.

By using coconut oil or any food that is a good source of MCTs, you will be able to avoid an accumulation of glucose in the blood because the ketone energy source replaces it.

Bad Fats

Now let's have a look at the good and the bad fats to see why they are so different.

In chapter 5, I briefly discussed the names of good and bad fats and mentioned to avoid:

Trans- and hydrogenated fats

What are they exactly?

Trans fat is a lipid fat molecule and can, in small amounts, occur naturally in certain foods such as meat and dairy products. Food manufacturers process this molecule widely. Following the hydrogenation, it becomes saturated fat. Processed trans fats are dangerous to us. I won't go into the science behind it because I would need to use terms such as "double bonds" and "hydrogen atoms" which would distract from the actual topic of the book. Studies show, though, that this type of fat is linked with an increased risk of coronary heart disease.

All this makes me wonder why food is treated this way in the first place.

The answers are good ones and difficult to argue against:

- *Because such a process helps to increase the shelf life of our foodstuff*

- *Hydrogenated oil can cook on a hotter setting for longer. And it won't get rancid as quickly as other oils.*

The fast food industry was practically built on processing techniques, which is only one of many reasons not to consume it.

Why is it bad for our health?

Trans fats have no nutritional value whatsoever. If that's not reason enough, then know that trans fats increase our bad cholesterol (LDL) rates. To make it a double whammy, it also lowers the good cholesterol (HDL) rates. That is worrying information, as it increases the risk of heart disease.

The National Academy of Sciences (NAS) recommends the consumption of trans fats be as low as possible.

Good Fats

This leaves us wondering which fats we *can* eat.

- Plant-based and fish-based fats and oils, which are poly-unsaturated and mono-unsaturated fats, are good. It seems the word "unsaturated," is the one to look out for when wanting to opt for healthier choices.

- These types of fats differ in the bonding of molecules. They help to keep the good HDL cholesterol rates up and the Bad LDL cholesterol levels down, thus decreasing your chances of heart disease.

You should consume

- **Olive oil**
- **Peanut oil**
- **Omega 3 oils**
- **Nuts and seeds**
- **Avocado**
- **Leaf vegetables**

Saturated fats should still be an essential part of your diet though. If eaten in moderation, they can help raise HDL (good cholesterol) levels. Plus, it can also change the bad cholesterol into a more benign form, making it less harmful. Saturated fats can be found in various natural foods in small quantities. For instance:

- **Butter**
- **Red meats like beef and lamb**
- **Poultry skin**
- **Cheese**
- **Cream**

Fats also produce energy, so if you have a low-fat diet, you could find yourself suffering from lethargy. Some fatty acids are in fact needed to help build up our immune system. The increased metabolism assists in the buildup of muscle mass. Also, because fat does not digest quickly, it gives us that "full" feeling, so you are likely to eat less.

Chapter 8 - Meal Ideas and Macro Counting

<u>Macronutrients</u>
This is an ideal way to measure your intake of food. You will still need to know what your daily calorie intake should be and then balance out the macronutrients accordingly.

There are the 3 main food types that provide the human body with all its nutrients: carbs, protein and fat. They are known as macronutrients. These nutrients are the building blocks for our dietary intake and will provide us with energy.

First, you need to set your own calorie goal, which is based on your size, age and gender. Remember, you want to be burning more energy than you are consuming.

Here's a rough idea of the amount of macro-based foods you should be eating as part of your daily calorie intake on a keto diet:

10% of your daily calorie intake should come from carbohydrates, 20-30% from proteins and 60-70% from good fats.

For example, if you choose 30% protein, then your fat intake should be 60%.

By dividing your food types into macronutrients, you are giving yourself a healthy dietary balance. It also prevents you from overusing certain food types. As a result, your digestive system will cope better.

Below you will find suggestions for well-balanced meals:

Breakfast

Cheesy Sausage
1 oz. low carb sausage (always check for sugar and salt content)
1 cup of your favorite bell pepper, sliced and roasted in 1 tbsp. olive oil
1 oz. grated cheese
You can melt the cheese on top or simply top with cold grated cheese

This comes out to around 530 calories, the micronutrient count of which is 9g carbs, 23g protein, and 45g fat.

Bacon and Eggs
2 pieces of back bacon
2 eggs fried in 1 tbsp. of butter or olive oil
Dry-fry the bacon; any bacon fat is for the eggs

When ready, fry 3/4cup of fresh spinach and half a cup of mushrooms in the bacon fat. If there isn't enough bacon fat to do this, use a little from your egg-cooking portion.

This recipe comes at around 780 calories (carbs 5g, protein 25g, fat 56g). Note that the increase in carbs and fat have raised the caloric value.

Lunch

Corn Dog Muffins
This is a great recipe because the muffins will stay good for up to 5 days in a sealed container.

Combine 1 tbsp. butter and 1 tbsp. coconut oil, melted. Mix together 1 cup coconut flour, 1 cup almond flour, 6 whisked eggs, a pinch of salt, 1tsp baking soda, and the melted oils.

Stir in 10 organic hot dogs, sliced into small pieces.

Add 1 cup coconut milk and mix gently to make a batter. Don't overdo the mixing or the mixture will be too heavy.

This should make 22 muffins.

Bake in a preheated oven at 350F for 15 minutes.

Each muffin will be around 160 calories (carbs 2g, protein 6g, fat 13g).

Cheese Taco Rolls
Serves 3

Sprinkle 2 cups of grated cheddar cheese to cover a layer of greased parchment paper that is spread out in a flat baking tin. Don't layer the cheese too thinly or it will just crisp up.

Bake this in a hot oven for around 15 minutes or until browned. It is ready once you can slip a spatula underneath, and it feels a little loose.

Take out of the oven. Spread over the cooked cheese 1 cup of precooked ground meat that has been seasoned with Mexican spices, such as cumin, chili, and garlic.

Pop back into the oven to warm up meat for around 5-10 mins.

Remove from baking tin. Add your prepared cold toppings, such as chopped avocado, sliced tomatoes, onions, peppers, olives, or even lettuce.

Cut into 3 long pieces and roll each slice before it cools.

Macros for 500 calories per taco are: carbs 2g, fat 35g, protein 37g.

Chicken and Bacon Salad
Serves 2

Place a layer of sliced lettuce in a bowl.

Add chopped soft avocado and slices of grilled chicken breast.

Sprinkle with crispy bacon pieces.

Top with a couple of tbsp. of creamy Caesar salad dressing.

Macros per dish for 200 calories are: carb 8g, protein 24g, fat 34g.

Main Meal

Cheese Burger
Serves 2

Season 8 oz. ground beef to taste with spices such as Cajun or herbs such as parsley, oregano or basil and make 2 flat patties.

Cube 1 oz. mozzarella and slice 2 oz. of cheddar cheese. Place the cubed mozzarella cheese in the center of the patties and pull up the patty around the cheese to enclose it in the middle.

Fry one side of the patties in 1-2 tbsp. melted butter. When browned, turn over the patties and fry until cooked. Place the sliced cheddar cheese on top.

Once cooked, place precooked slice of bacon on each patty.

Eat warm with a serving of green vegetables or green salad of choice.

Macros per burger for 600 calories are: carbs 1.5g, protein 33g, fat 50g.

Chicken and Zucchini Noodles
Serves 4

Toss 2 lb. chopped free range chicken breast in a bowl; season with 1/4 tsp. ginger powder and 1/4 tsp. garlic powder, then salt and pepper to taste.

Fry in 2 tbsp. hot peanut oil for around 3-4 mins or until cooked, then remove from skillet.

Add 3 whisked eggs to skillet and scramble them, then remove from pan.

Add to skillet 1/2 cup organic chicken broth, 3 tbsp. peanut butter, 2 tbsp. tamari (or soy sauce), 1 tbsp. rice vinegar, 1/2 cup chopped scallion (spring onion or sliced onion), 2 crushed garlic cloves, and 1 tsp. red pepper flakes. Stir well and heat for 3 mins.

Add the chicken, 4 spiralized zucchinis, the scrambled eggs, and ½ cup beansprouts to the pan.

Stir together well and cook on heat for around 1 min.

Serve on plates.

Macros per serving for 700 calories are: carb 8g, protein 90g, fat 34g.

Low Carb Breads

Cloud Bread - Carb Free
Serves 10

Separate 3 eggs, keep both yolks and whites.

Whisk egg yolks.

Stir in 3 tbsp. full-fat cream cheese (any flavor you like, but not sweet), plus a pinch of salt, or 1 tbsp. sweetener, which helps reduce the taste of the tartar.

Sprinkle 1/4 tsp. cream of tartar into your egg whites and whisk until firm.

Carefully stir in egg yolk mixture.

Use a flat oven tray, layered with a baking sheet and sprayed with oil.

Spoon 10 equally sized portions on your cooking tray and bake for 30 mins on 300F.

Macros per serving for 35 calories are: carb 0.5g, protein 2.2g, fat 2.6g.

Almond Flour Microwaveable Bread Bun
Serves 1
Grease a microwaveable small dish, about the size of a cup, with a small blob of melted butter.
In a bowl, mix together:

- *35g almond flour*
- *1/4 tsp baking powder*
- *1 egg, whisked*
- *2 tbsp. of either olive oil OR melted coconut oil OR melted butter*
- *Small pinch of salt*

Pour the mixture into your greased container, and cook for 1 minute on high.
Empty the contents of the cup onto a saucer and put back in the microwave to cook on high for another 30 seconds. Doing this will help the bread to cook more evenly.
Macros per serving for 130 calories are: carb 3g, protein 2g, fat 13g.
You can use more quantities and bake whole bread loaves. No one said you had to do without bread!

Chapter 9 - Meal Planning for Beginners

If you have chosen not to follow the IF path as a quick way to attain ketosis, then don't worry - you can still do it with the keto diet alone. For a beginner, it can be quite daunting, and without the IF, it will take a little longer to get into ketosis. Cutting down on carbs and sticking to the keto diet will get you there. This chapter will provide some useful tips for those starting out.

Ketosis without Fasting

Start on a very low-carb plan for the first 3 days by not eating more than 20g net carbs daily.
To make sure you're going in the right direction, this might be a good time to use "Ketostix." These are test strips that indicate the level of ketones in your urine. They are simple to use; just dip them into urine in a bottle or place under the stream when urinating.

Keeping track of your dietary intake is important at this point in order to reduce the risk of illness. If you recall, I spoke about the imbalance in electrolytes that occurs when your body begins to use fats for energy instead of glucose (sugars from the carbs). You must drink plenty of fluids and maybe even add a little extra salt to your food. At this point, taking potassium, sodium or magnesium supplements along with a vitamin C supplement could be beneficial. This is because you are not used to this dietary intake and may not be getting enough nutrients. Don't worry, you will learn what suits your body as time goes on.

The feelings you may experience when altering your diet can be similar to detoxing.

The beginning can be difficult. You may have cravings, headaches, and all those other symptoms I mentioned in chapter 4. Don't worry, all is not lost - they will pass, and it will be worth it.

Put together a meal plan before you start. It will make your introduction to keto easier to manage. Also think about time management to make sure you are on target. It will take away the need to calculate things when you're not feeling your best.

Remember your macros and balance those carbs, proteins, and fats.

Ideas for Meal Planning

<u>Breakfasts:</u>
- Pancakes, made with eggs and cream cheese (add a little almond flour if you don't like the texture.)
- Eggs
- Bacon
- Sausage
- Check the ingredients and avoid any added fillers such as rusk
- Be careful of the ingredients in vegetarian sausages. Avoid those that have a high grain and sugar content. Don't worry about the salt at this stage – you need it!
- Mushrooms
- Tomatoes
- Cloud Bread (see the recipe in chapter 7.)

<u>Lunches:</u>
- Use cream cheese pancakes to roll sandwich ingredients inside, such as ham, cheese, egg, and mayo
- Salads with ingredients such as, lettuce, cucumber, bell peppers, radish, tomatoes
- You can add ingredients such as, tuna, cheese, or eggs to your salads

- Sprinkle seeds on your salad to add a crunchy texture

<u>Dinners:</u>
Meats:
- Chicken drum sticks
- Chicken breast with soy sauce and sesame seeds
- Fish, such as salmon or cod
- Pork chops
- Ground beef
- Beef steaks

Vegetables:
- Cauliflower
- Green leafy vegetables such as spinach, bok choy, or chard

Sauces:
- Add extra shredded cheese to cream cheese, then melt together to make a rich sauce
- Use Worcestershire, soy sauce, or mustard to add flavor to your sauces and gravies

<u>Snacks:</u>
- Beef or chicken broth
- Avocado
- Around 10 nuts

- Unprocessed string cheese

Drinks:
- Coffee with full-fat cream
- Green tea
- Water with lemon slices
- If you sweeten your drinks, use an alternative natural sweetener such as Stevia or Erythritol
- Red wine in the recommended moderation - you will need to deduct this from your carb count for the day

Other Tips for Low-Carb Meals

- For cooking, use olive, coconut oil, or butter.
- Make soups from bell pepper, cauliflower, chicken, or broccoli and add cream if you want
- Replace cereal-based flour with almond or coconut flour to make low-carb bread
- Cauliflower rice is quite filling and soaks up the flavor of sauces.
- Shredded zucchini or shredded carrots are a great replacement for pasta.
- Cabbage leaves make great wraps - steam them for a few minutes and then add your preferred ingredients.

- Introduce 1-2 squares of dark chocolate into your diet as an occasional treat.
- Chopped jalapenos add a hot burst of flavor to many dishes.
- Make your own salad dressings using balsamic vinegar, olive oil, then add herbs and spices that you like
- Thicken sauces with flax meal or xanthine gum.
- Cream is great for sauces, including sour cream or plain yogurt.
- Use parmesan cheese for a crunchy topping or coating.
- Most meats are fine to eat, but watch out for any sugar content in processed meats such as sausages and bacon
- Make your own burgers and meatballs, but don't use breadcrumbs
- Crustless quiches are a great addition to a salad
- Make your own vegetable patties, using lentils to blend the ingredients together.
- Learn how to make up a good low-carb muesli using nuts, seeds and coconut shavings.
- Homemade is best and helps avoid the processed food pitfalls.

You can gradually increase your carb intake, from the original 20g up to 50g per day, but do it over a few weeks.

- After 3 days go to 30g
- Week 2 - 40g
- Week 3 - 50g
- Stay at 50g if you can - it is a comfortable zone to maintain permanently for ketosis
- If you need to come out of ketosis, you can increase to 100g for a short while

Chapter 10 - Exercises for Toning Up During Weight Loss

Using only exercise to lose weight is not ideal, unless you are prepared to do extensive daily workouts whereby you burn up lots of energy and carbs. However, exercise is great way to keep the body healthy in other ways. Even if you are dieting or changing your eating habits to include my recommended IF and low-carb way of eating, you should still have a basic exercise routine. You are doing your heart a big favor and toning up muscles and any excess loose skin from your weight loss.

When I talk about toning, I do not mean having a perfectly sculptured body. I am talking about basic health needs. If you are losing a lot of weight, you will most likely have to deal with loose skin. The toning up I am referring to has more to do with looking and feeling better.

Leaner Muscles

You will find that certain areas of your body need a little extra help when you are losing weight. To help tighten up that loose skin, you need to strengthen the muscles in those areas. It does not need to involve heavy weight training, just a regular routine 2-3 times a week. Let's start out with a little stretching routine:

Legs

- Lay down on your side
- Prop up your body, using the elbow that is on the floor
- The leg on the floor should be stretched out straight
- Now that you are in position, raise the leg that is not on the floor until you feel it pull on your inner thigh
- Stay in that position and count to 5
- Repeat 10 times
- Now turn over to the other side and repeat the whole process

Arms

- Sit somewhere comfortable with your back straight, but supported.
- Your arms need to be able to hang down at your sides, so an armless chair is good for this exercise.
- Hold a dumbbell in each hand and raise your arms so they are straight in front of you, weights on the inside
- If you don't have dumbbells, use food tins instead
- Lift your arms slowly above your head
- Bend the elbows so the weights are behind your ears
- Stay in that position and count to 5
- Repeat the whole process 10 times

Abdomen

- Lay on your back with your feet flat on the floor and knees bent
- Put your hands behind your neck and lock your fingers together

- Try to use your hands to help lift your head and shoulders off the floor, but don't bend the neck
- You should be feeling the pull in your stomach muscles
- To do the "crunch" more effectively, aim at raising your upper back from the floor
- Stay in that position and count to 5
- Repeat the whole process 10 times

Neck

There's nothing worse than being left with a double chin, when you're losing weight. Here's an easy exercise to help loosen those flabby jowls.

- Stand up or sit down, with your arms hanging at your side
- Move your head back, so you are now looking upwards. If you feel a bad pain in your neck, stop and go no further with this exercise
- Open your jaws as wide as you can
- Slowly close them, pushing out your bottom jaw a little to pull on your chin
- Stay in that position and count to 5
- Repeat the exercise 10 times

These are just some simple stretching exercises to get you started. Strength training and stretching are the best exercises you can do for toning up. Try and complete this or a similar routine of exercises every other day at least.

- Find exercises that you can feel are stretching those main muscles. You should always feel a gentle pull on your muscles. If you're not, then it's time to increase the weight or make the exercise harder. Congratulate yourself at this stage - you're beginning to tone up those unused muscles and tighten any loose skin.

- Always stay hydrated, especially when exercising

- Your skin needs all the nutrients it can get to help the process, so eat plenty of omega 3 foods and consume plenty of those good fats.

- Perform at least 3 stretching exercises 3 or more times a week.

- Once you are up and running with a good exercise routine, move on to add cardiovascular exercises too. Go jogging or take a walk. Riding your bike or swimming are also good choices. Anything that gets your heart rate up for short periods of time, really.

Conclusion

You have to take care of your body; it's the only one you got. After all, if you feel good, then who knows what you can achieve in your life.

This is a guide to help you make the right choices for yourself. I wanted to show you how a certain way of eating can make you feel healthier and content with life. To achieve this goal, I have discussed the benefits of Intermittent Fasting as well as a low-carb, ketogenic diet. It is only fair to inform you of the possible side effects. In the beginning you will sometimes feel unwell, but such effects are also short-lived. However, carefully balancing your meals can prevent the side effects altogether. Such a drastic change in diet and lifestyle can be difficult in the beginning. This guide will take you through the difficulties that you may encounter. If you fall off the path in the beginning, don't worry, newbies often do. Once you're seasoned, you will be glad you made the changes. Your body will be thanking you for it, as you feel more energetic and suffer fewer health problems.

You can, of course, choose only one of the options I've talked about. If you introduce Intermittent Fasting to your lifestyle, perhaps later, you can look at adding the keto diet. Should you decide this is the way for you, then remember you must always eat healthy meals. Balancing your diet well is vital for success.

Planning ahead is the key to good management. At first, it may seem like there aren't enough foods that you're allowed to eat. But if you sit down and plan your meals, you will soon come to realize that there are plenty of ingredients in the low-carb way of life. I could write you a whole cook book on low carb recipes, alone. Once you start looking, you will find lots of delicious meal ideas.

Even if you're vegetarian, you can make IF and the keto diet work. Nuts will certainly play a major role if you decide to give it a go. Vegetarians can get their good fats from nuts rather than meat. Pecans, almonds, Brazil nuts, pine nuts, hazelnuts, walnuts and macadamias are just some of the choices there are. Some nuts, such as cashews, can be high in carbs, so be aware when balancing your macros. Protein will be the biggest challenge, especially if you do not eat dairy. Nuts and seeds will help, though, and if necessary you could use a protein supplement.

This guide is just that. It is intended to guide you through the ups and downs of IF and keto. I hope I have convinced you that it can and does lead to a healthier and happier lifestyle. It will take a while to find the foods you like and come up with delicious recipes. Once you get to that stage, consider home-cooking in bulk. That way, you are not tempted to dash out and buy the wrong types of food when in a hurry.

We are all guilty of rushing through life, as though every day is the last one. We rush around at work, often commuting to get there. Even leisure time passes so fast that we can barely fit in the activities we enjoy. Consider slowing down once in a while and take a little time for yourself. Take a little timeout and make a plan to:

- Find your favorite recipes
- Cook in bulk so you can freeze meals
- Exercise for toning up and tightening loose skin while you lose weight
- Find cardio exercises will help to keep your heart healthy

I hope I managed to illustrate how important it is to acquire good eating habits and keep them. Look after your body as much as you can – it's the first step to a long and healthy life.

Thank you so much for your support through buying and reading this book, it means the world to me!

If you never want to miss out on one of my future books, consider signing up for my newsletter here

http://bit.ly/allannewsletter

and checking out my author's page here

http://amzn.to/allanmccampbell

-Allan

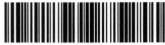

Made in the USA
Columbia, SC
13 March 2018